MEASUREMENTS

DATE: ______________

MAN BOOBS	
WAIST	
SHOULDERS	
UPPER ARM	
FOREARM	
CALF	
WEIGHT	

Date :

Breakfast

Lunch

Dinner

Extras

(A)　　　　　　　　(B)

Treats	1	2	3	4	5	6	7	8	9	10	11	12	13	14	15	16	17	18	19	20

Log

Vegetables ○ ○ ○ ○ ○ ○ ○
Fruit ○ ○ ○ ○ ○ ○ ○
Water ○ ○ ○ ○ ○ ○ ○

Notes

Goal-Digging List

Date :

Breakfast

Lunch

Dinner

Extras

(A)

(B)

Treats	1	2	3	4	5	6	7	8	9	10	11	12	13	14	15	16	17	18	19	20

Log

Vegetables ○ ○ ○ ○ ○ ○ ○

Fruit ○ ○ ○ ○ ○ ○ ○

Water ○ ○ ○ ○ ○ ○ ○

Notes

Goal-Digging List

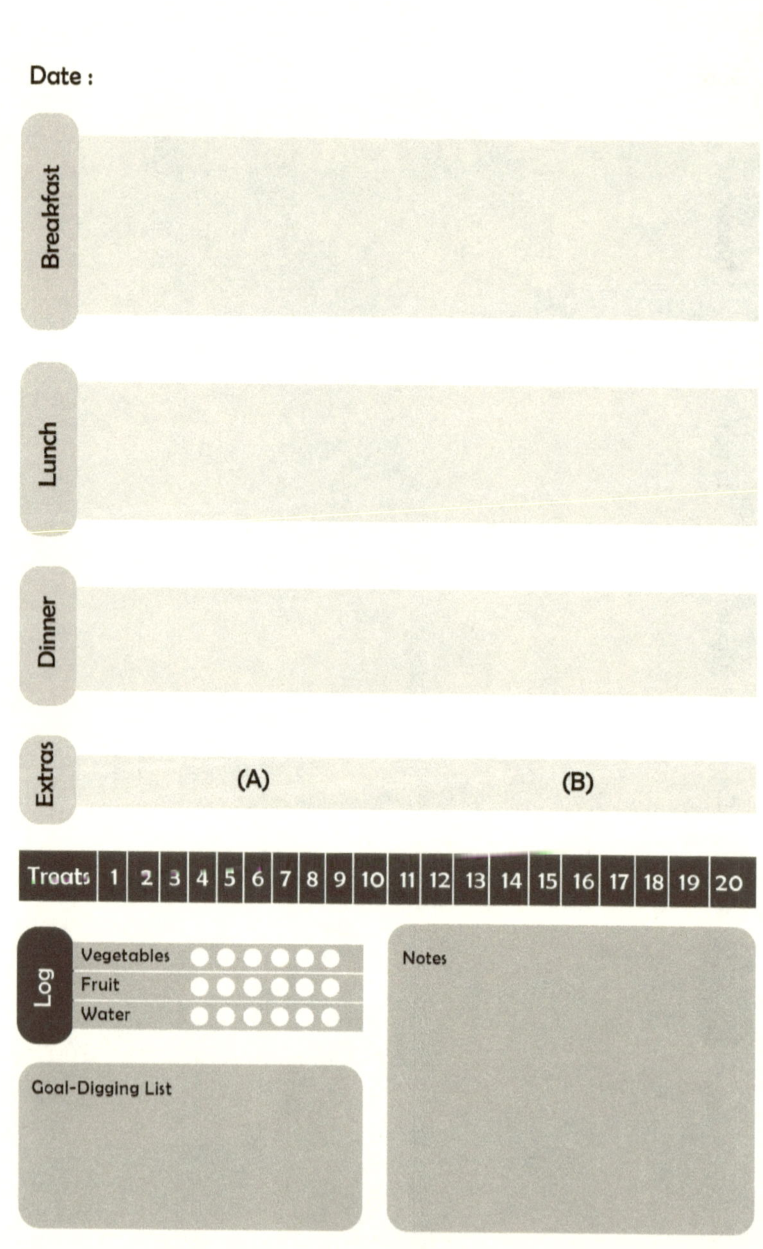

Date :
Breakfast
Lunch
Dinner
Extras
(A)
(B)
Treats 1 2 3 4 5 6 7 8 9 10 11 12 13 14 15 16 17 18 19 20
Log
Vegetables
Fruit
Water
Notes
Goal-Digging List

Date :

Breakfast

Lunch

Dinner

Extras

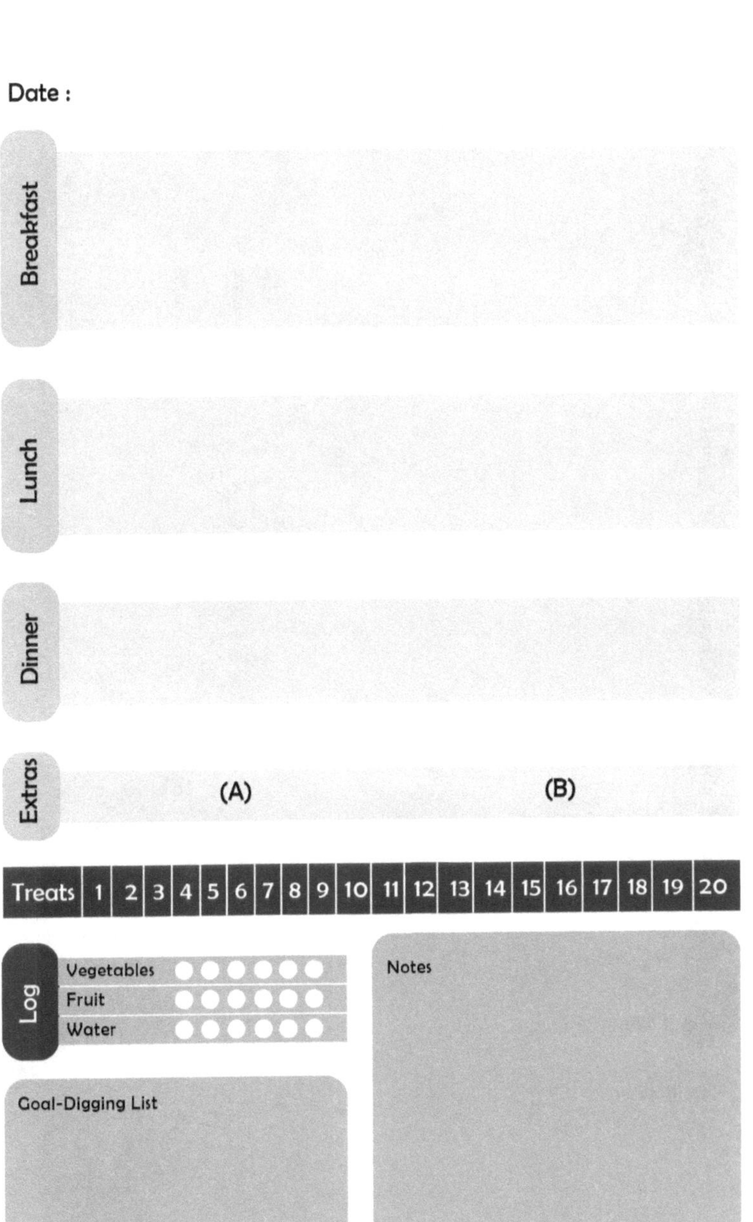

Date :

Breakfast

Lunch

Dinner

Extras

(A)   (B)

Treats	1	2	3	4	5	6	7	8	9	10	11	12	13	14	15	16	17	18	19	20

Log

Vegetables ○ ○ ○ ○ ○ ○
Fruit ○ ○ ○ ○ ○ ○
Water ○ ○ ○ ○ ○ ○

Notes

Goal-Digging List

Date :

Breakfast

Lunch

Dinner

Extras

(A)   (B)

Treats	1	2	3	4	5	6	7	8	9	10	11	12	13	14	15	16	17	18	19	20

Log

Vegetables

Fruit

Water

Notes

Goal-Digging List

Date :

Breakfast

Lunch

Dinner

Extras

(A) (B)

Treats	1	2	3	4	5	6	7	8	9	10	11	12	13	14	15	16	17	18	19	20

Log

Vegetables

Fruit

Water

Notes

Goal-Digging List

WORKOUT LOG

NAME:_________________________ GOALS:_________________________

EXERCISES	SETS	REPS	WT	REST	TIME	1 RM	NOTES

DATE:_________ WEIGHT:_________ SLEEP:_________ CALORIES:_________

EXERCISES	SETS	REPS	WT	REST	TIME	1 RM	NOTES

DATE:_________ WEIGHT:_________ SLEEP:_________ CALORIES:_________

EXERCISES	SETS	REPS	WT	REST	TIME	1 RM	NOTES

DATE:_________ WEIGHT:_________ SLEEP:_________ CALORIES:_________

EXERCISES	SETS	REPS	WT	REST	TIME	1 RM	NOTES

DATE:_________ WEIGHT:_________ SLEEP:_________ CALORIES:_________

EXERCISES	SETS	REPS	WT	REST	TIME	1 RM	NOTES

DATE:_________ WEIGHT:_________ SLEEP:_________ CALORIES:_________

TV *show*

NAME:
SEASONS:
EPISODES:

SEASON:

THE ENDING

-Thoughts-

Rating: ☆ ☆ ☆ ☆ ☆

MEASUREMENTS

DATE: _______________

| MAN BOOBS |
| WAIST |
| SHOULDERS |
| UPPER ARM |
| FOREARM |
| CALF |
| WEIGHT |

Date :

Breakfast

Lunch

Dinner

Extras

(A)　　　　　　　　　(B)

Treats	1	2	3	4	5	6	7	8	9	10	11	12	13	14	15	16	17	18	19	20

Log

Vegetables ○○○○○○

Fruit ○○○○○○

Water ○○○○○○

Notes

Goal-Digging List

Date :

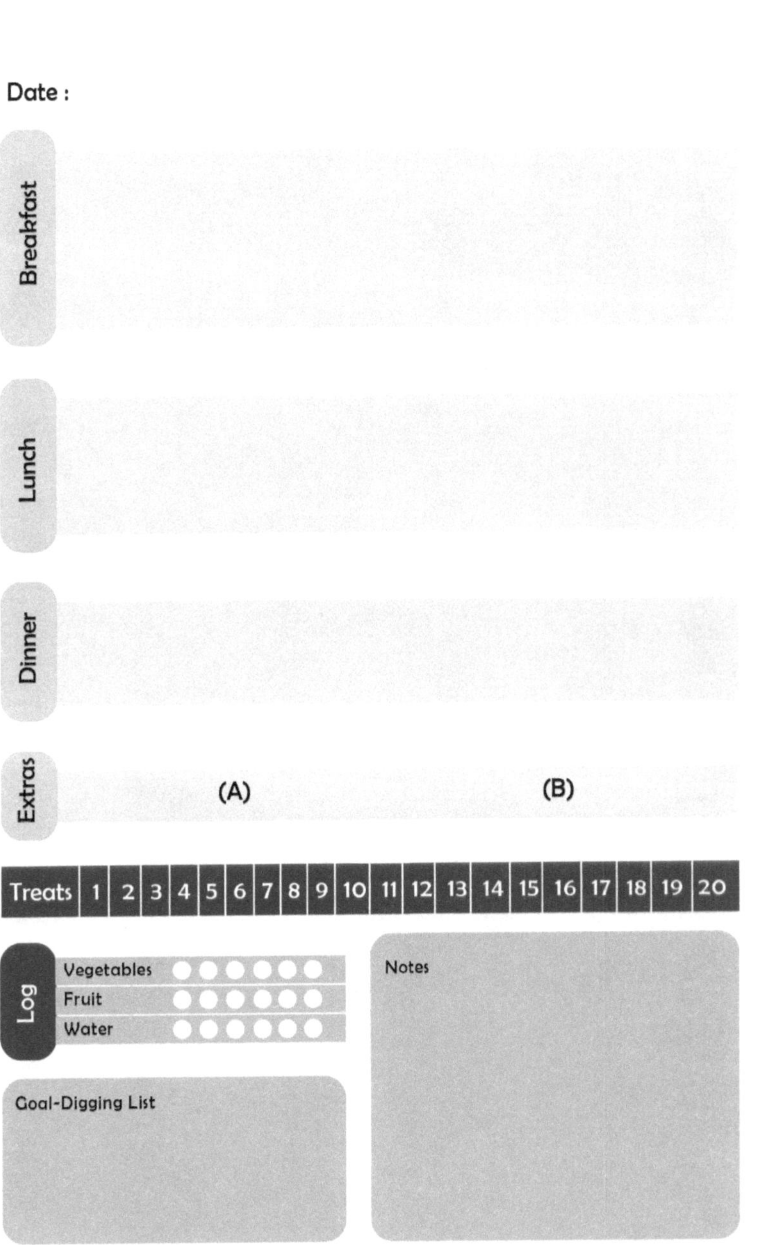

Date :

Breakfast

Lunch

Dinner

Extras

(A)   (B)

Treats	1	2	3	4	5	6	7	8	9	10	11	12	13	14	15	16	17	18	19	20

Log
Vegetables
Fruit
Water

Notes

Goal-Digging List

Date :

Breakfast

Lunch

Dinner

Extras

(A)   (B)

Treats	1	2	3	4	5	6	7	8	9	10	11	12	13	14	15	16	17	18	19	20

Log

Vegetables ○ ○ ○ ○ ○ ○

Fruit ○ ○ ○ ○ ○ ○

Water ○ ○ ○ ○ ○ ○

Notes

Goal-Digging List

Date :

Breakfast

Lunch

Dinner

Extras

(A)   (B)

Treats	1	2	3	4	5	6	7	8	9	10	11	12	13	14	15	16	17	18	19	20

Log

Vegetables ⭘⭘⭘⭘⭘⭘

Fruit ⭘⭘⭘⭘⭘⭘

Water ⭘⭘⭘⭘⭘⭘

Notes

Goal-Digging List

Date :

Breakfast

Lunch

Dinner

Extras

(A)   (B)

Treats	1	2	3	4	5	6	7	8	9	10	11	12	13	14	15	16	17	18	19	20

Log

Vegetables ○ ○ ○ ○ ○ ○ ○

Fruit ○ ○ ○ ○ ○ ○ ○

Water ○ ○ ○ ○ ○ ○ ○

Notes

Goal-Digging List

Date :

Breakfast

Lunch

Dinner

Extras

(A)

(B)

Treats	1	2	3	4	5	6	7	8	9	10	11	12	13	14	15	16	17	18	19	20

Log

Vegetables

Fruit

Water

Notes

Goal-Digging List

WORKOUT LOG

NAME:____________________________ GOALS:____________________________

EXERCISES	SETS	REPS	WT	REST	TIME	1 RM	NOTES

DATE:_________ WEIGHT:_________ SLEEP:_________ CALORIES:_________

EXERCISES	SETS	REPS	WT	REST	TIME	1 RM	NOTES

DATE:_________ WEIGHT:_________ SLEEP:_________ CALORIES:_________

EXERCISES	SETS	REPS	WT	REST	TIME	1 RM	NOTES

DATE:_________ WEIGHT:_________ SLEEP:_________ CALORIES:_________

EXERCISES	SETS	REPS	WT	REST	TIME	1 RM	NOTES

DATE:_________ WEIGHT:_________ SLEEP:_________ CALORIES:_________

EXERCISES	SETS	REPS	WT	REST	TIME	1 RM	NOTES

DATE:_________ WEIGHT:_________ SLEEP:_________ CALORIES:_________

TV *show*

NAME:
SEASONS:
EPISODES:

SEASON:

THE ENDING

-Thoughts-

Rating: 

MEASUREMENTS

DATE: _______________

MAN BOOBS	
WAIST	
SHOULDERS	
UPPER ARM	
FOREARM	
CALF	
WEIGHT	

Date :

Breakfast

Lunch

Dinner

Extras

(A)   (B)

Treats	1	2	3	4	5	6	7	8	9	10	11	12	13	14	15	16	17	18	19	20

Log

Vegetables	○ ○ ○ ○ ○ ○ ○ ○
Fruit	● ● ● ● ● ● ●
Water	● ● ● ● ● ● ●

Notes

Goal-Digging List

Date :

Breakfast

Lunch

Dinner

Extras

(A)

(B)

Treats	1	2	3	4	5	6	7	8	9	10	11	12	13	14	15	16	17	18	19	20

Log

Vegetables

Fruit

Water

Notes

Goal-Digging List

Date :

Breakfast

Lunch

Dinner

Extras

(A)   (B)

Treats	1	2	3	4	5	6	7	8	9	10	11	12	13	14	15	16	17	18	19	20

Log

Vegetables ○ ○ ○ ○ ○ ○

Fruit ○ ○ ○ ○ ○ ○

Water ○ ○ ○ ○ ○ ○

Notes

Goal-Digging List

Date :

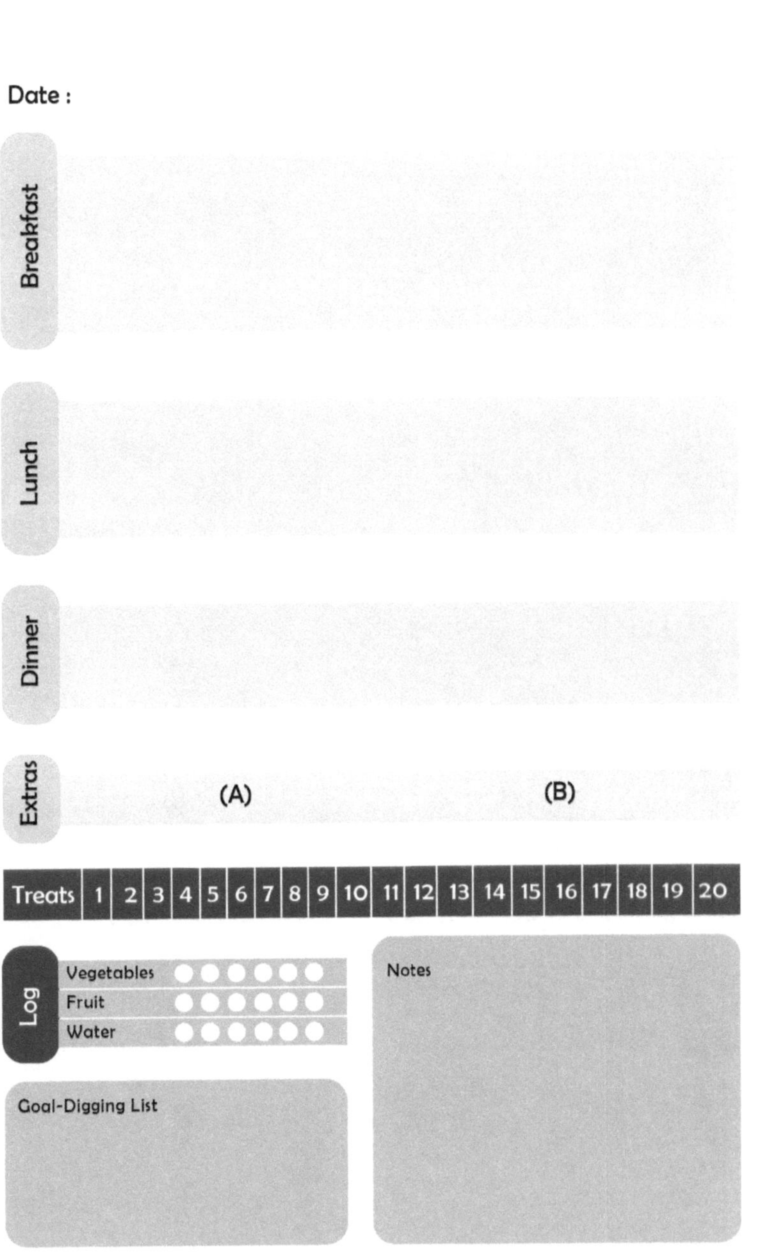

Date :

Breakfast

Lunch

Dinner

Extras   (A)   (B)

Treats	1	2	3	4	5	6	7	8	9	10	11	12	13	14	15	16	17	18	19	20

Log

Vegetables

Fruit

Water

Notes

Goal-Digging List

Date :

Breakfast

Lunch

Dinner

Extras

(A)   (B)

Treats	1	2	3	4	5	6	7	8	9	10	11	12	13	14	15	16	17	18	19	20

Log

Vegetables ○ ○ ○ ○ ○ ○

Fruit ○ ○ ○ ○ ○ ○

Water ○ ○ ○ ○ ○ ○

Notes

Goal-Digging List

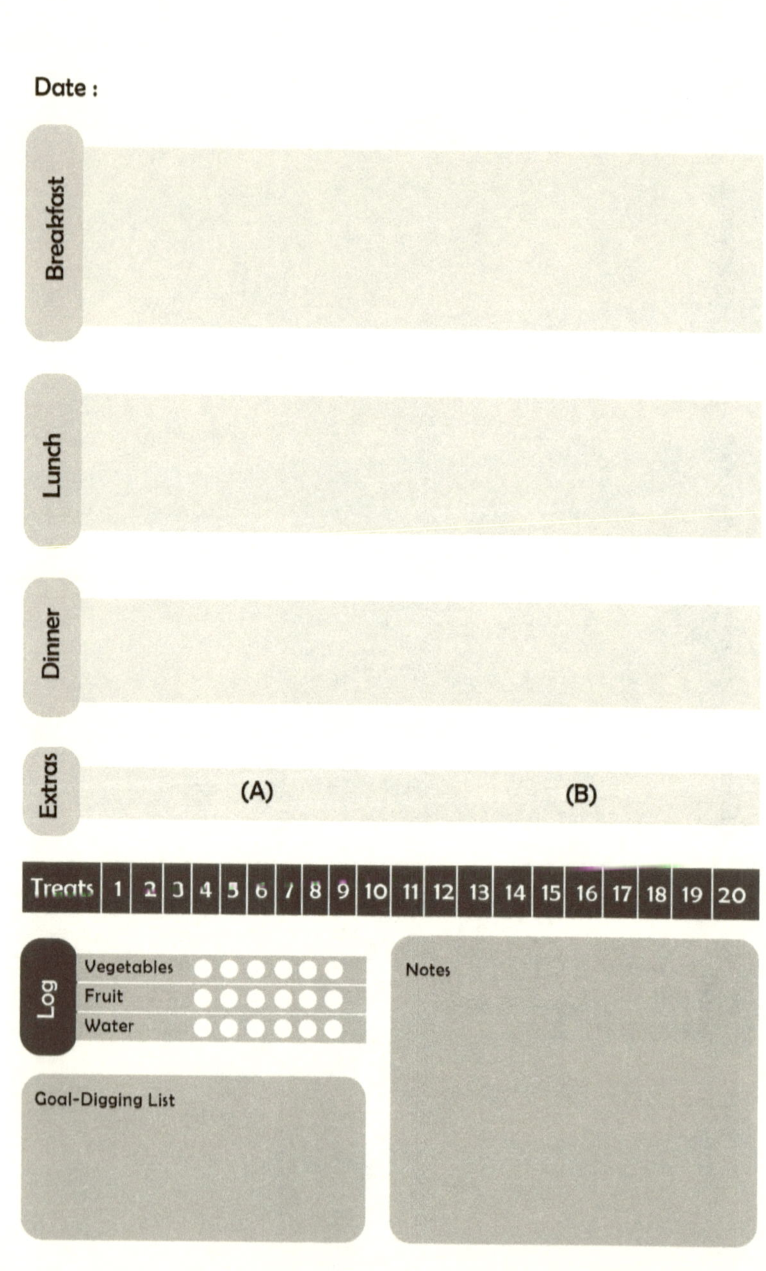Date :
Breakfast
Lunch
Dinner
Extras
(A)
(B)
Treats 1 2 3 4 5 6 7 8 9 10 11 12 13 14 15 16 17 18 19 20
Log
Vegetables
Fruit
Water
Notes
Goal-Digging List

WORKOUT LOG

NAME:_______________________   GOALS:_______________________

EXERCISES	SETS	REPS	WT	REST	TIME	1 RM	NOTES

DATE:_________   WEIGHT:_________   SLEEP:_________   CALORIES:_________

EXERCISES	SETS	REPS	WT	REST	TIME	1 RM	NOTES

DATE:_________   WEIGHT:_________   SLEEP:_________   CALORIES:_________

EXERCISES	SETS	REPS	WT	REST	TIME	1 RM	NOTES

DATE:_________   WEIGHT:_________   SLEEP:_________   CALORIES:_________

EXERCISES	SETS	REPS	WT	REST	TIME	1 RM	NOTES

DATE:_________   WEIGHT:_________   SLEEP:_________   CALORIES:_________

EXERCISES	SETS	REPS	WT	REST	TIME	1 RM	NOTES

DATE:_________   WEIGHT:_________   SLEEP:_________   CALORIES:_________

TV 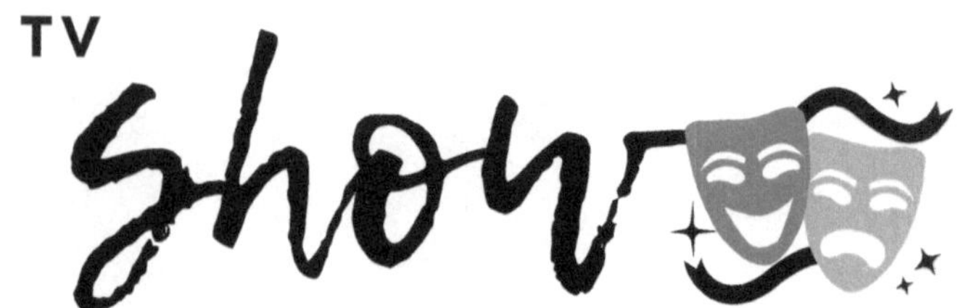

NAME:
SEASONS:
EPISODES:

SEASON:

THE ENDING

-Thoughts-

Rating:     

MEASUREMENTS

DATE: _______________

MAN BOOBS	
WAIST	
SHOULDERS	
UPPER ARM	
FOREARM	
CALF	
WEIGHT	

Date :

Breakfast

Lunch

Dinner

Extras

(A)   (B)

Treats	1	2	3	4	5	6	7	8	9	10	11	12	13	14	15	16	17	18	19	20

Log

Vegetables ○○○○○○
Fruit ○○○○○○
Water ○○○○○○

Notes

Goal-Digging List

Date :

Breakfast

Lunch

Dinner

Extras

(A) (B)

Treats	1	2	3	4	5	6	7	8	9	10	11	12	13	14	15	16	17	18	19	20

Log

Vegetables ○ ○ ○ ○ ○ ○
Fruit ○ ○ ○ ○ ○ ○
Water ○ ○ ○ ○ ○ ○

Notes

Goal-Digging List

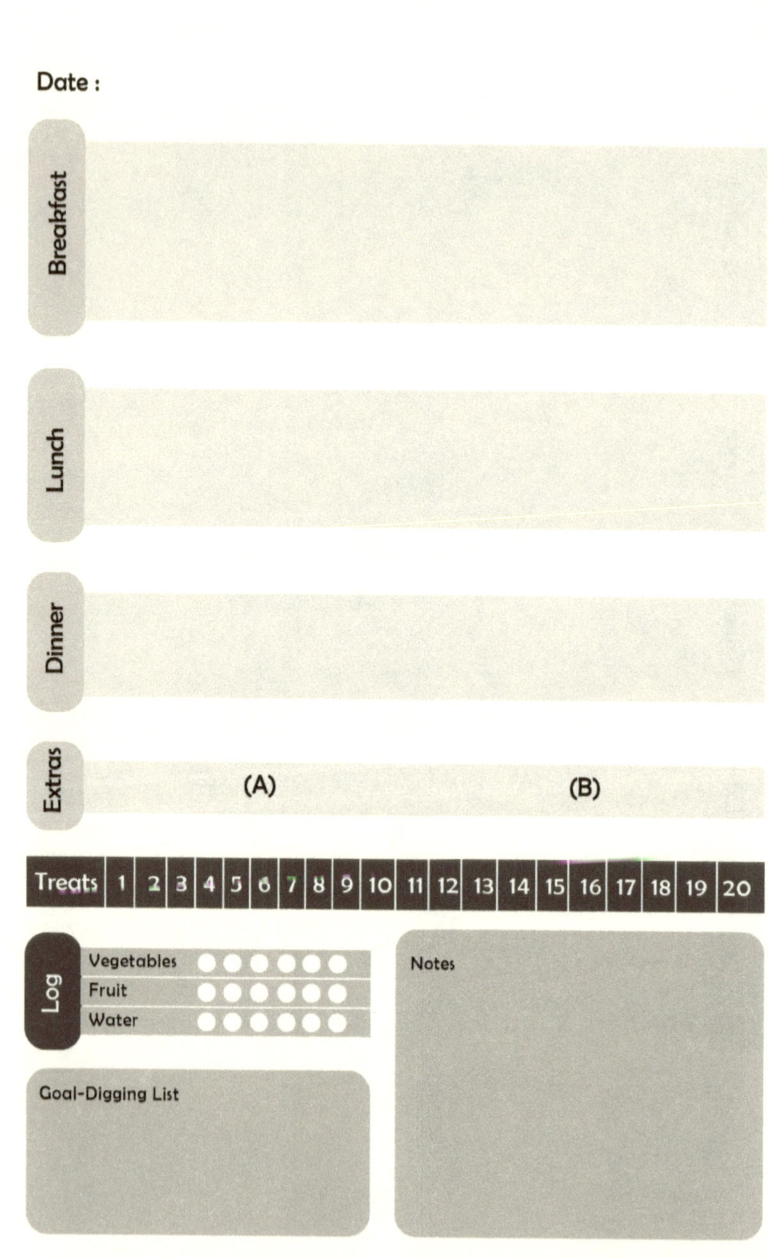

Date :
Breakfast
Lunch
Dinner
Extras
(A)
(B)
Treats
1 2 3 4 5 6 7 8 9 10 11 12 13 14 15 16 17 18 19 20
Log
Vegetables
Fruit
Water
Notes
Goal-Digging List

Date :

Breakfast

Lunch

Dinner

Extras
(A)   (B)

Treats	1	2	3	4	5	6	7	8	9	10	11	12	13	14	15	16	17	18	19	20

Log

Vegetables

Fruit

Water

Notes

Goal-Digging List

Date :

Breakfast

Lunch

Dinner

Extras

(A)   (B)

Treats	1	2	3	4	5	6	7	8	9	10	11	12	13	14	15	16	17	18	19	20

Log

Vegetables ○○○○○○
Fruit ○○○○○○
Water ○○○○○○

Notes

Goal-Digging List

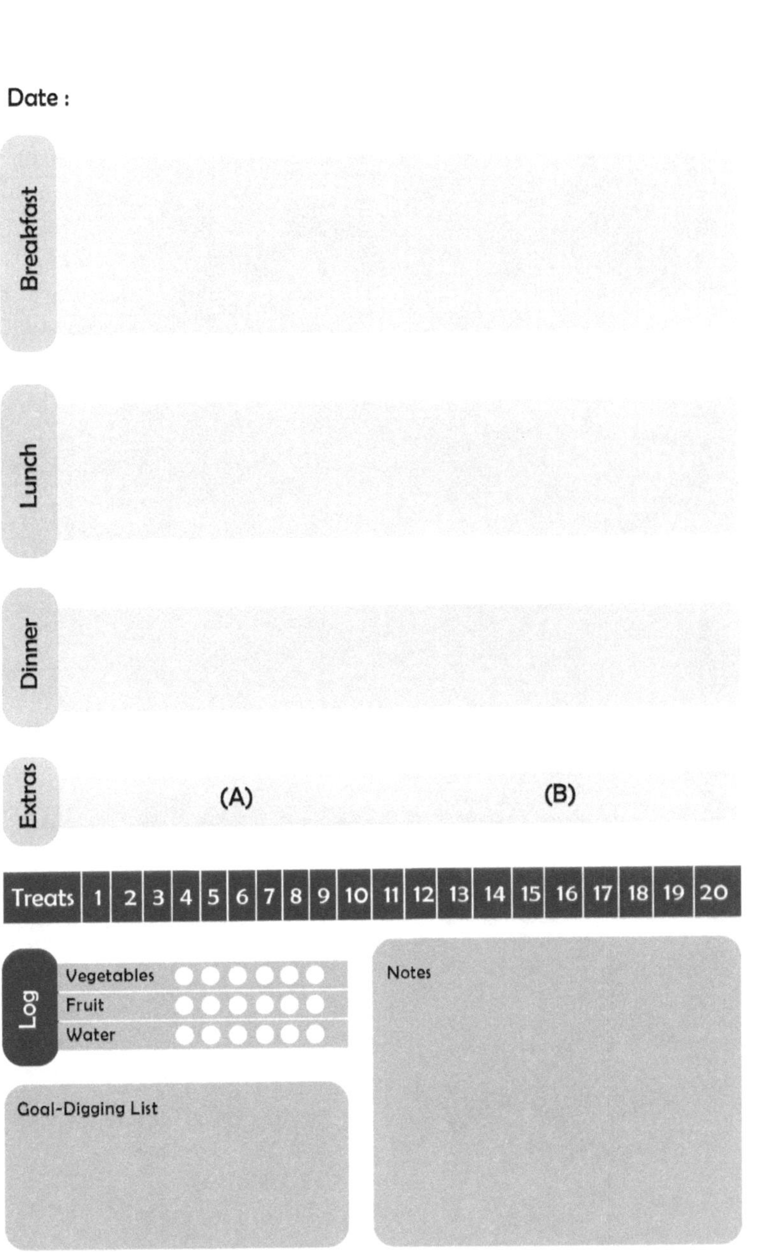

Date :
Breakfast
Lunch
Dinner
Extras
(A)
(B)
Treats 1 2 3 4 5 6 7 8 9 10 11 12 13 14 15 16 17 18 19 20
Log
Vegetables
Fruit
Water
Notes
Goal-Digging List

Date :

Breakfast

Lunch

Dinner

Extras

(A)   (B)

Treats	1	2	3	4	5	6	7	8	9	10	11	12	13	14	15	16	17	18	19	20

Log

Vegetables

Fruit

Water

Notes

Goal-Digging List

WORKOUT LOG

NAME:_________________________ GOALS:_________________________

EXERCISES	SETS	REPS	WT	REST	TIME	1 RM	NOTES

DATE:_________ WEIGHT:_________ SLEEP:_________ CALORIES:_________

EXERCISES	SETS	REPS	WT	REST	TIME	1 RM	NOTES

DATE:_________ WEIGHT:_________ SLEEP:_________ CALORIES:_________

EXERCISES	SETS	REPS	WT	REST	TIME	1 RM	NOTES

DATE:_________ WEIGHT:_________ SLEEP:_________ CALORIES:_________

EXERCISES	SETS	REPS	WT	REST	TIME	1 RM	NOTES

DATE:_________ WEIGHT:_________ SLEEP:_________ CALORIES:_________

EXERCISES	SETS	REPS	WT	REST	TIME	1 RM	NOTES

DATE:_________ WEIGHT:_________ SLEEP:_________ CALORIES:_________

TV
show

NAME:
SEASONS:
EPISODES:

SEASON:

THE ENDING

-Thoughts-

Rating: ☆ ☆ ☆ ☆ ☆

MEASUREMENTS

DATE:

Date :

Breakfast

Lunch

Dinner

Extras

(A)   (B)

Treats	1	2	3	4	5	6	7	8	9	10	11	12	13	14	15	16	17	18	19	20

Log

Vegetables ○ ○ ○ ○ ○ ○
Fruit ○ ○ ○ ○ ○ ○ ○
Water ○ ○ ○ ○ ○ ○ ○

Notes

Goal-Digging List

Date :

Breakfast

Lunch

Dinner

Extras   (A)   (B)

Treats	1	2	3	4	5	6	7	8	9	10	11	12	13	14	15	16	17	18	19	20

Log

Vegetables ○○○○○○
Fruit ○○○○○○
Water ○○○○○○

Notes

Goal-Digging List

Date :

Breakfast

Lunch

Dinner

Extras

(A)	(B)

Treats	1	2	3	4	5	6	7	8	9	10	11	12	13	14	15	16	17	18	19	20

Log

Vegetables ○ ○ ○ ○ ○ ○
Fruit ○ ○ ○ ○ ○ ○
Water ○ ○ ○ ○ ○ ○

Notes

Goal-Digging List

Date :

Breakfast

Lunch

Dinner

Extras

(A)   (B)

Treats	1	2	3	4	5	6	7	8	9	10	11	12	13	14	15	16	17	18	19	20

Log

Vegetables

Fruit

Water

Notes

Goal-Digging List

Date :

Breakfast

Lunch

Dinner

Extras

(A) (B)

Treats	1	2	3	4	5	6	7	8	9	10	11	12	13	14	15	16	17	18	19	20

Log

Vegetables	○ ○ ○ ○ ○
Fruit	○ ○ ○ ○ ○
Water	○ ○ ○ ○ ○

Notes

Goal-Digging List

Date :

Breakfast

Lunch

Dinner

Extras

(A)

(B)

Treats	1	2	3	4	5	6	7	8	9	10	11	12	13	14	15	16	17	18	19	20

Log

Vegetables

Fruit

Water

Notes

Goal-Digging List

Date :

Breakfast

Lunch

Dinner

Extras   (A)   (B)

Treats	1	2	3	4	5	6	7	8	9	10	11	12	13	14	15	16	17	18	19	20

Log

Vegetables

Fruit

Water

Notes

Goal-Digging List

WORKOUT LOG

NAME:_________________________ GOALS:_________________________

EXERCISES	SETS	REPS	WT	REST	TIME	1 RM	NOTES

DATE:_________   WEIGHT:_________   SLEEP:_________   CALORIES:_________

EXERCISES	SETS	REPS	WT	REST	TIME	1 RM	NOTES

DATE:_________   WEIGHT:_________   SLEEP:_________   CALORIES:_________

EXERCISES	SETS	REPS	WT	REST	TIME	1 RM	NOTES

DATE:_________   WEIGHT:_________   SLEEP:_________   CALORIES:_________

EXERCISES	SETS	REPS	WT	REST	TIME	1 RM	NOTES

DATE:_________   WEIGHT:_________   SLEEP:_________   CALORIES:_________

EXERCISES	SETS	REPS	WT	REST	TIME	1 RM	NOTES

DATE:_________   WEIGHT:_________   SLEEP:_________   CALORIES:_________

NAME:
SEASONS:
EPISODES:

SEASON:

THE ENDING

-Thoughts-

Rating: 

MEASUREMENTS

DATE:

MAN BOOBS

WAIST

SHOULDERS

UPPER ARM

FOREARM

CALF

WEIGHT

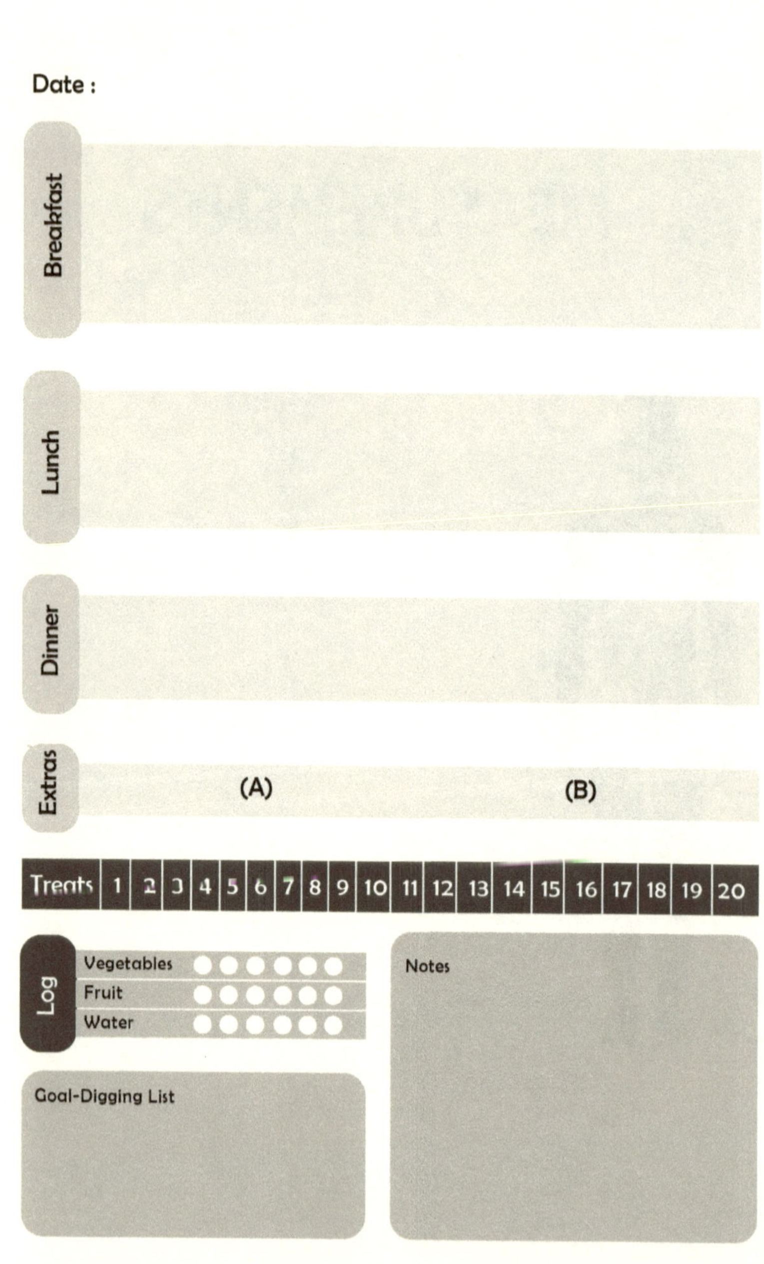

Date :
Breakfast
Lunch
Dinner
Extras
(A)
(B)
Treats
1 2 3 4 5 6 7 8 9 10 11 12 13 14 15 16 17 18 19 20
Log
Vegetables
Fruit
Water
Notes
Goal-Digging List

Date :

Breakfast

Lunch

Dinner

Extras

(A)   (B)

Treats	1	2	3	4	5	6	7	8	9	10	11	12	13	14	15	16	17	18	19	20

Log

Vegetables ○○○○○○○
Fruit ○○○○○○○
Water ○○○○○○○

Notes

Goal-Digging List

Date :

Breakfast

Lunch

Dinner

Extras

(A)   (B)

Treats	1	2	3	4	5	6	7	8	9	10	11	12	13	14	15	16	17	18	19	20

Log

Vegetables ○ ○ ○ ○ ○ ○

Fruit ○ ○ ○ ○ ○ ○

Water ○ ○ ○ ○ ○ ○

Notes

Goal-Digging List

Date :

Breakfast

Lunch

Dinner

Extras   (A)   (B)

Treats	1	2	3	4	5	6	7	8	9	10	11	12	13	14	15	16	17	18	19	20

Log

Vegetables ○○○○○○
Fruit ○○○○○○
Water ○○○○○○

Notes

Goal-Digging List

Date :

Breakfast

Lunch

Dinner

Extras

(A)   (B)

Treats	1	2	3	4	5	6	7	8	9	10	11	12	13	14	15	16	17	18	19	20

Log

Vegetables ○ ○ ○ ○ ○ ○ ○ ○

Fruit ○ ○ ○ ○ ○ ○ ○ ○

Water ○ ○ ○ ○ ○ ○ ○ ○

Notes

Goal-Digging List

Date :

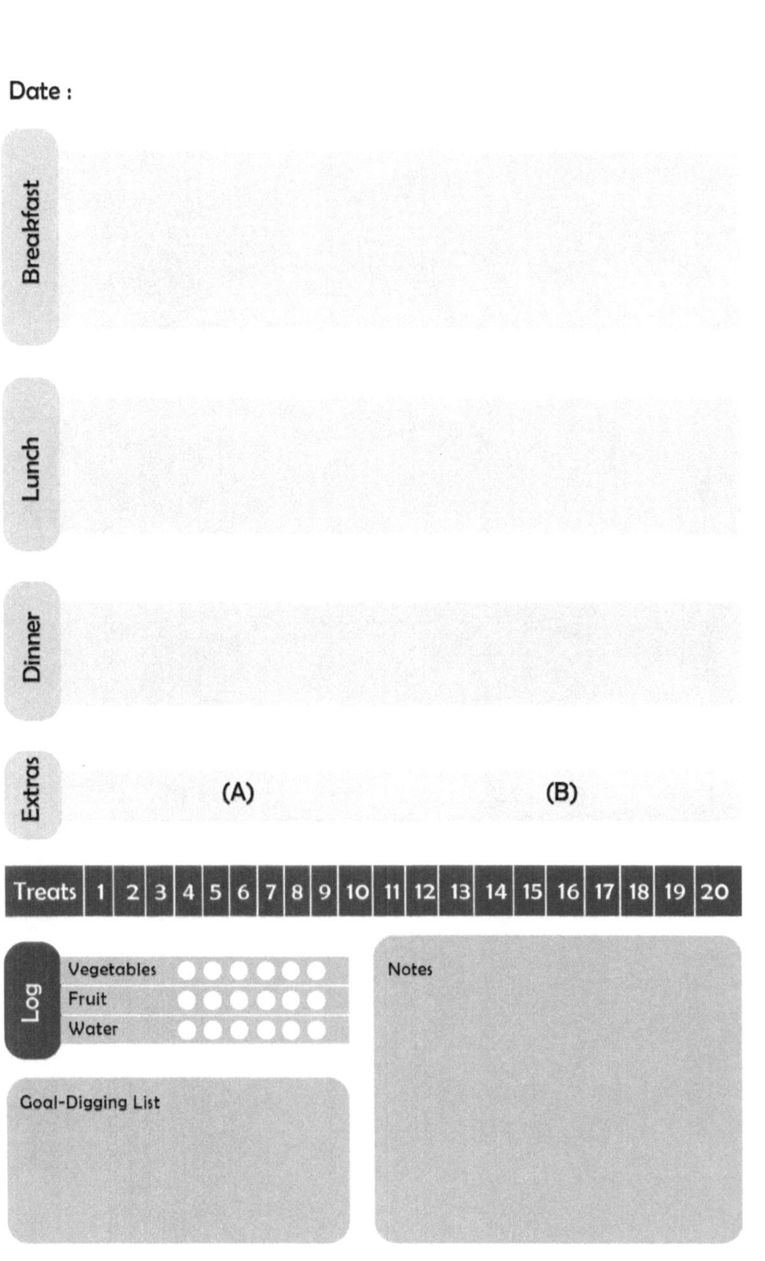

Date :

Breakfast

Lunch

Dinner

Extras

(A)   (B)

Treats	1	2	3	4	5	6	7	8	9	10	11	12	13	14	15	16	17	18	19	20

Log

Vegetables

Fruit

Water

Notes

Goal-Digging List

WORKOUT LOG

NAME:_________________________ GOALS:_________________________

EXERCISES	SETS	REPS	WT	REST	TIME	1 RM	NOTES

DATE:_________ WEIGHT:_________ SLEEP:_________ CALORIES:_________

EXERCISES	SETS	REPS	WT	REST	TIME	1 RM	NOTES

DATE:_________ WEIGHT:_________ SLEEP:_________ CALORIES:_________

EXERCISES	SETS	REPS	WT	REST	TIME	1 RM	NOTES

DATE:_________ WEIGHT:_________ SLEEP:_________ CALORIES:_________

EXERCISES	SETS	REPS	WT	REST	TIME	1 RM	NOTES

DATE:_________ WEIGHT:_________ SLEEP:_________ CALORIES:_________

EXERCISES	SETS	REPS	WT	REST	TIME	1 RM	NOTES

DATE:_________ WEIGHT:_________ SLEEP:_________ CALORIES:_________

NAME:
SEASONS:
EPISODES:

SEASON:

THE ENDING

Rating:     

KETOGENIC FOODS

MEATS	VEGGIES	VEGGIES	FRUITS
Beef	Avocado	Cucumber	Blackberries
Sausage	Asparagus	Chards	Cranberries
Bacon	Argula	Bell Peppers	Blueberries
Lamb	Broccoli	Green Beans	Lemon
Pork	Cauliflower	Collards	Lime
Veal	Brussel Sprouts	Mushrooms	Raspberries
Chicken/Turkey	Cabbage	Spinach	Strawberries
Eggs	Celery	Olives	Plantains (paleo)

DAIRY	CONDIMENTS	OILS & FATS	HERBS & SPICES
Cheese (all kinds)	Balsamic Vinegar	Avocado Oil	Garlic
Sour Cream	Beef/Chicken Broth	Butter	Salt & Pepper
Cream Cheese	Bonito Flakes	Coconut Butter	Oregano
Heavy Cream	Tartar Sauce (keto)	Duck Fat	Paprika
Greek Yogurt	Dijon Mustard	Lard/Ghee	Cumin
Almond Milk	Mayo	Nut Oils	Chili Pepper
Cashew Milk	Low Sugar Ketchup	Olive Oil	Basil
Coconut Cream	Pickles	Pork Rinds	Ginger

BAKING	FISH/SEAFOOD	DRINKS	MISC.
Almond Flour	Anchovy	Diet Soda (moderation)	Canned Tuna
Almond Meal	Haddock / Cod	Coffee	Pesto
Cashew Flour	Halibut	Tea	Soy Sauce
Oat Fiber	Crab/Lobster	Gatorade Zero	Aioli
Psyllium Husk	Mackerel	Protein Shake	Béarnaise
Whey Protein	Salmon	Club Soda	Vinaigrette
Flax meal	Tuna	Broth	Hot Sauce
Hazelnut Flour	Red Snapper	Coconut Water	Guacamole

NOTES:

LOW CARB GROCERY IDEAS

FRESH PRODUCE

☐ Asparagus	☐ Cauliflower	☐ Onions
☐ Avocado	☐ Celery	☐ Radishes
☐ Bell Peppers	☐ Cucumber	☐ Salad Mix
☐ Berries	☐ Eggplant	☐ Squash
☐ Broccoli	☐ Fennel	☐ Tomatoes
☐ Brussel Sprouts	☐ Garlic	☐ Bok Choi
☐ Cabbage	☐ Green Beans	☐ Chives
☐ Carrots	☐ Mushrooms	☐ Spinach

MEAT AND SEAFOOD

☐ Bacon	☐ Lamb	☐ Fish
☐ Beef	☐ Pork	☐ Crab
☐ Bison	☐ Rotisserie Chicken	☐ Lobster
☐ Chicken	☐ Sausage	☐ Scallops
☐ Deli meat	☐ Turkey	☐ Shrimp
☐ Ground Beef / Ground Turkey	☐ Oyster	☐ Mussels

DAIRY PRODUCTS

☐ Butter	☐ Eggs	☐ Sour Cream
☐ Cheese	☐ Greek Yogurt, full fat	☐ Ghee
☐ Cream Cheese	☐ Heavy Whipping Cream	☐ Mayo

PANTRY ITEMS

☐ Avocado oil	☐ Tea/Coffee	☐ Moon Cheese
☐ Beef Jerky	☐ Pork Rinds	☐ Low Carb Protein Bars
☐ Bone Broth	☐ Mayonnaise	☐ All Natural Peanut Butter
☐ Tuna, Salmon (canned)	☐ Low Carb Salad Dressing	☐ Stevia
☐ Coconut Butter	☐ Olive oil, extra virgin	☐ Almonds
☐ Coconut Oil	☐ Olives	☐ Spices
☐ Almond Milk	☐ Sweeteners	☐ Almond Flour

FROZEN / OTHER

☐	☐	☐
☐	☐	☐
☐	☐	☐
☐	☐	☐

LOW CARB SHOPPING LIST

FRESH PRODUCE

MEAT AND SEAFOOD

DAIRY PRODUCTS

PANTRY ITEMS

FROZEN / OTHER

LOW CARB SHOPPING LIST

FRESH PRODUCE

MEAT AND SEAFOOD

DAIRY PRODUCTS

PANTRY ITEMS

FROZEN/OTHER

LOW CARB SHOPPING LIST

FRESH PRODUCE

MEAT AND SEAFOOD

DAIRY PRODUCTS

PANTRY ITEMS

FROZEN / OTHER

LOW CARB SHOPPING LIST

FRESH PRODUCE

MEAT AND SEAFOOD

DAIRY PRODUCTS

PANTRY ITEMS

FROZEN/OTHER

LOW CARB SHOPPING LIST

FRESH PRODUCE

MEAT AND SEAFOOD

DAIRY PRODUCTS

PANTRY ITEMS

FROZEN / OTHER

LOW CARB SHOPPING LIST

FRESH PRODUCE

MEAT AND SEAFOOD

DAIRY PRODUCTS

PANTRY ITEMS

FROZEN/OTHER

RUNNING / JOGGING LOG

YEAR _________ MONTH _________

DATE	DISTANCE	TIME	PACE	HR	REST HR	RUN TYPE	SHOES	NOTES

www.ingramcontent.com/pod-product-compliance
Lightning Source LLC
Chambersburg PA
CBHW051227250726
48655CB00006B/2634